# LITTLE MONSTERS,
## it's time to go to bed!

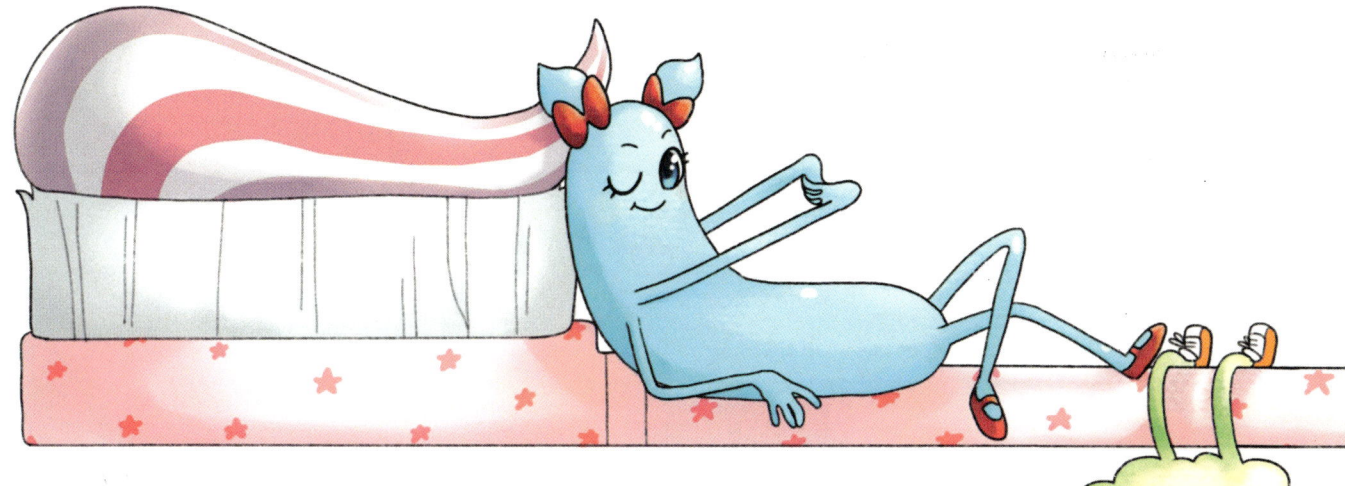

How to put little monsters to sleep
with a toothbrush and dental floss

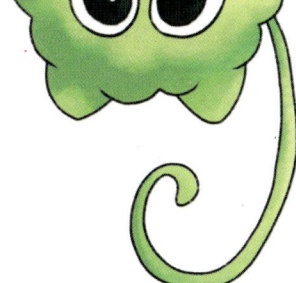

by Olivia Longray

It was beginning to get dark outside. Time to go to bed.

Betsy had already put her toy bear and her doll to bed. They had played all day and were very tired.

"Now we just need to put the little monsters to bed," mother said.

"Monsters? What monsters?" Betsy was surprised.

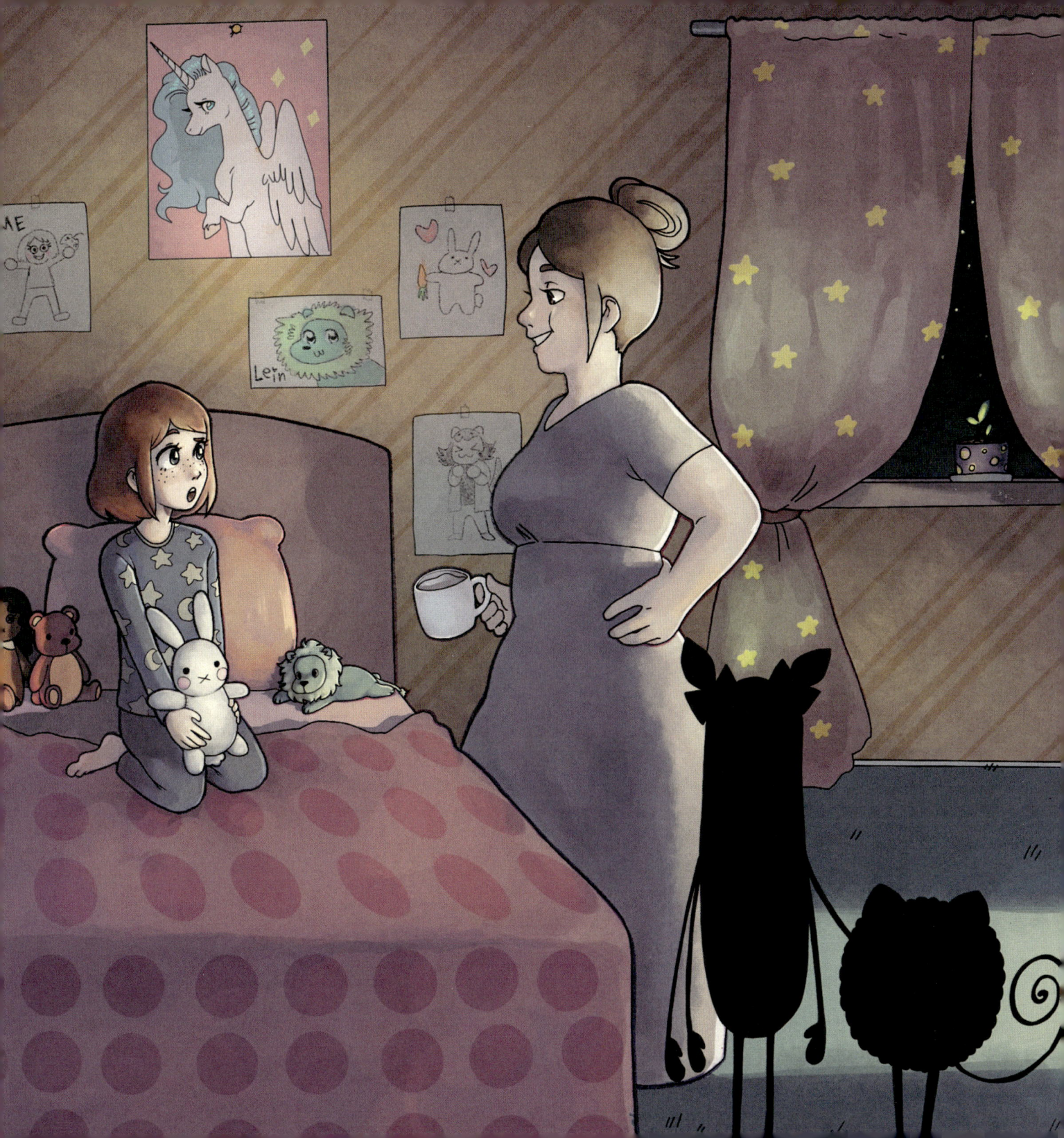

All the toys in the room looked at each other in surprise. There were no monsters among them, but mother knew that they existed.

"They are tiny bacteria that live in the mouth of every human being. They are very active," mother explained.

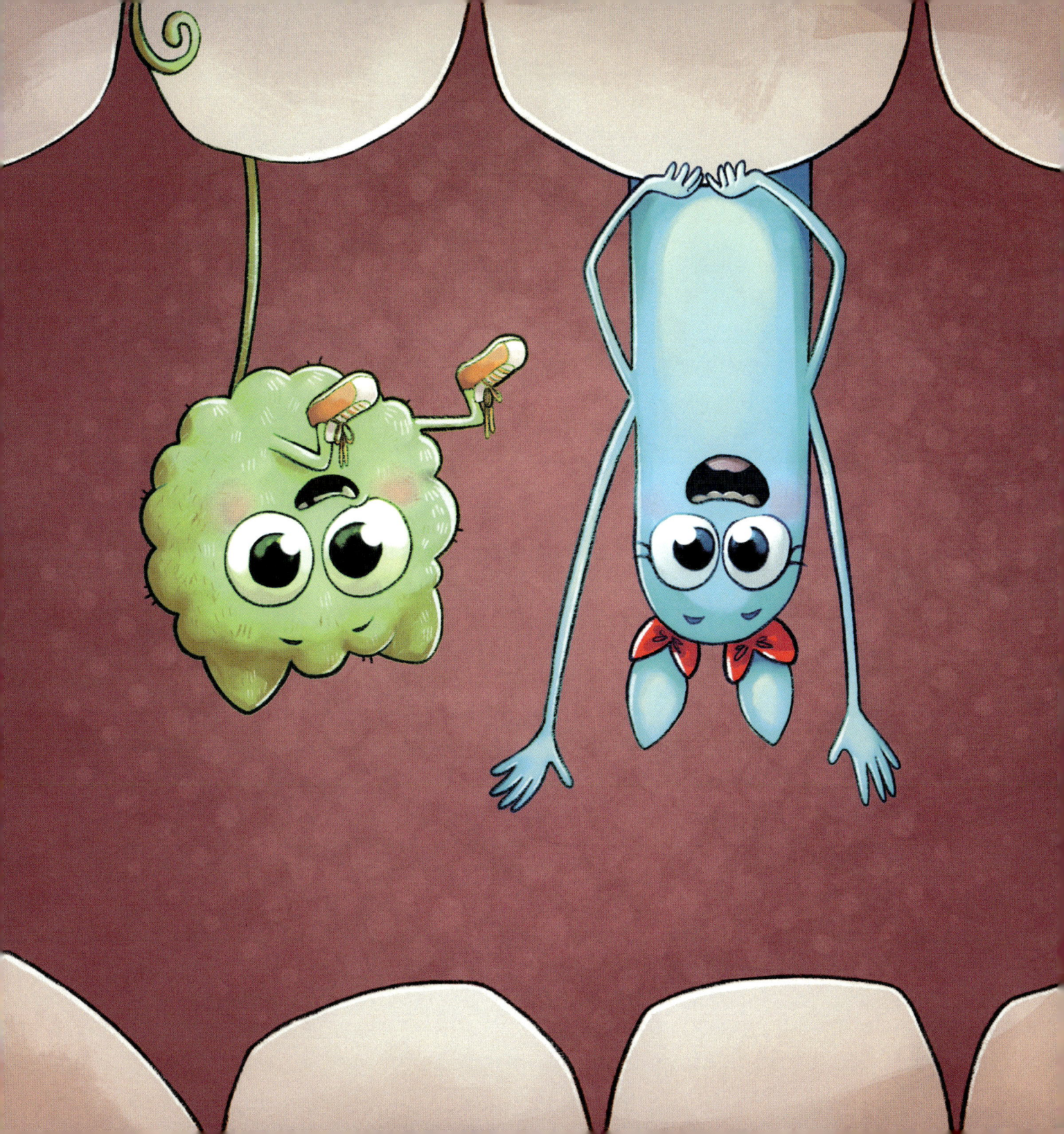

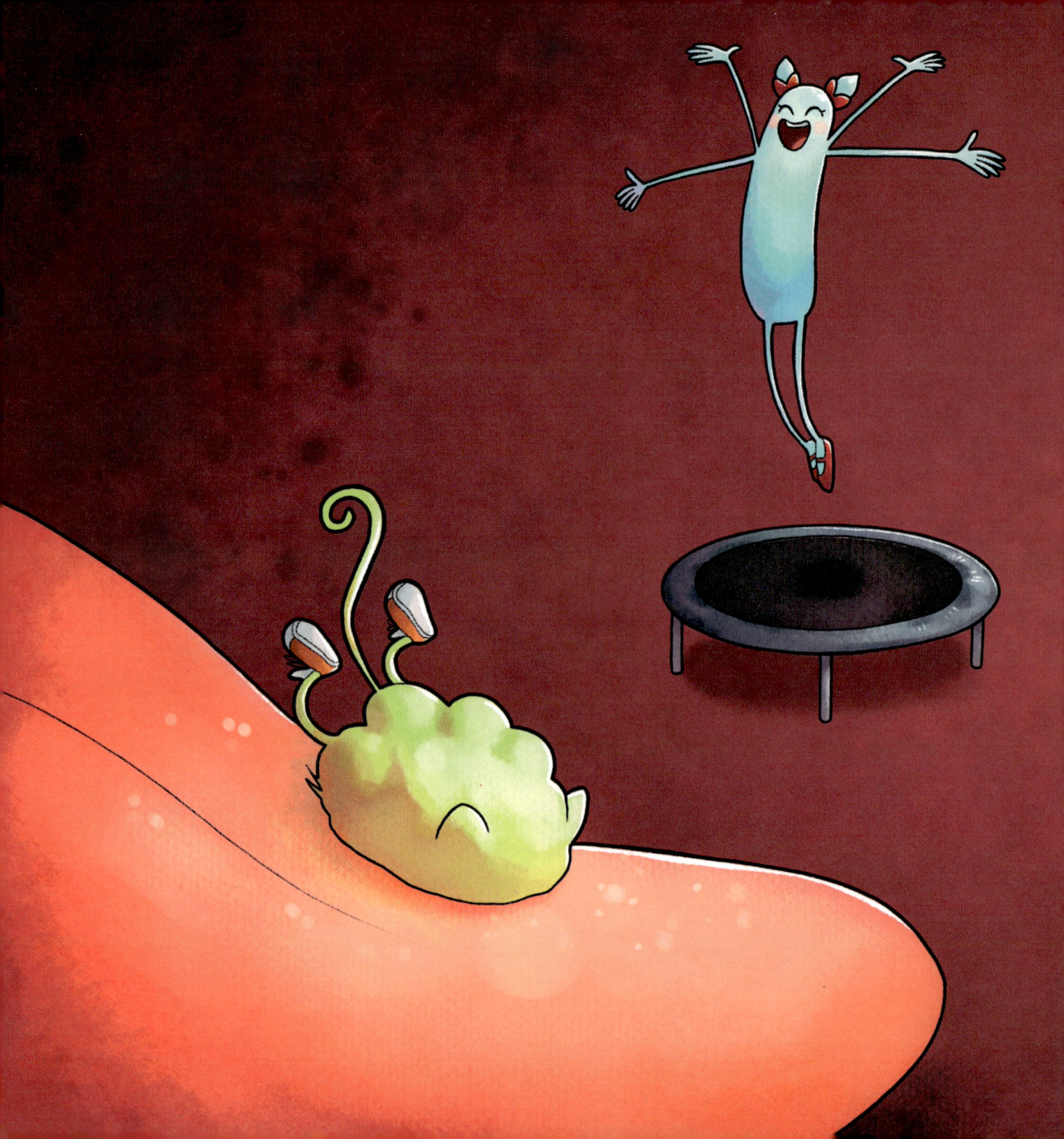

Betsy listened closely to see if she could hear anybody moving around in her mouth. Meanwhile, monster Toothy and monster Mouthy's games were in full swing.

Toothy slid down the tongue, as if sliding down a hill, while Mouthy jumped on trampolines. She placed them in the mouth, one near each cheek, and jumped up to the ceiling, or rather, to the palate, touching it with her hands.

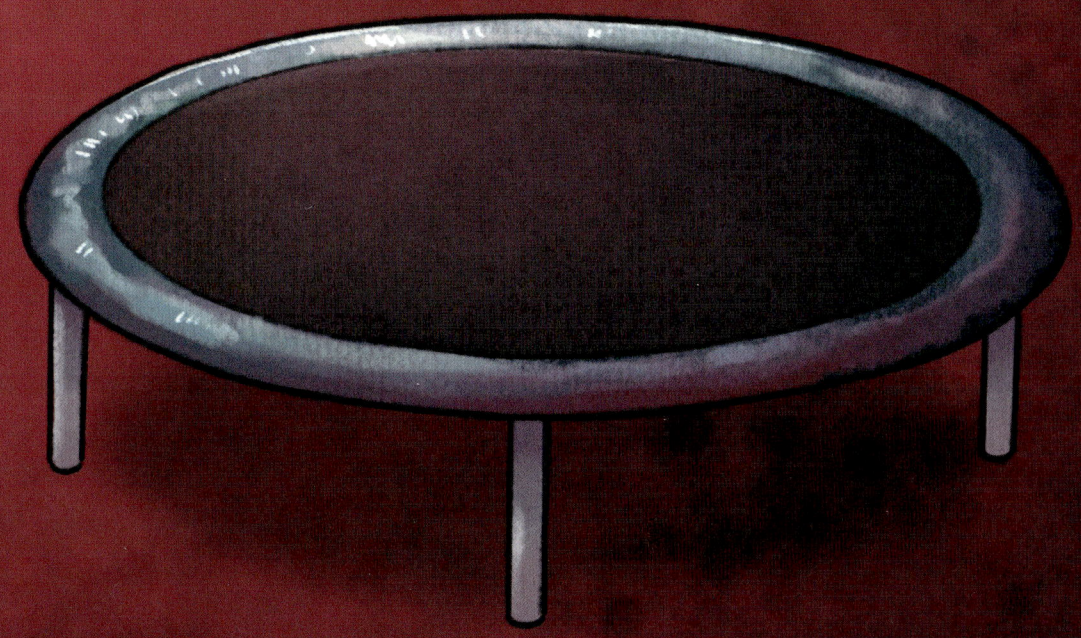

"My monsters do not want to go to bed at all," said Betsy.

"Well, mine are already asleep," mother whispered. She had brushed her teeth with a minty toothpaste, and the monsters immediately started to fall sleep. Now these strange creatures in her mouth were dreaming of mint candy.

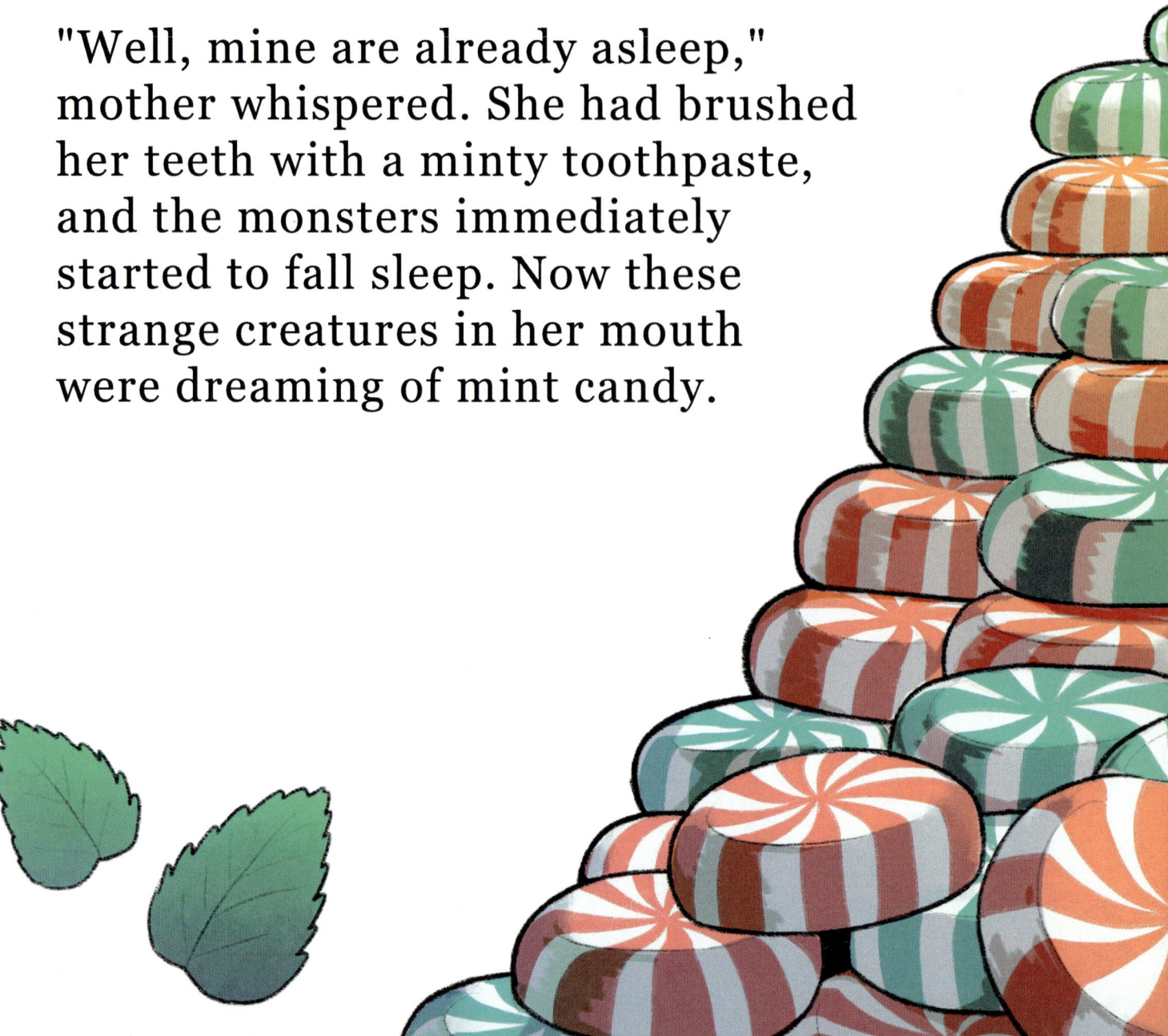

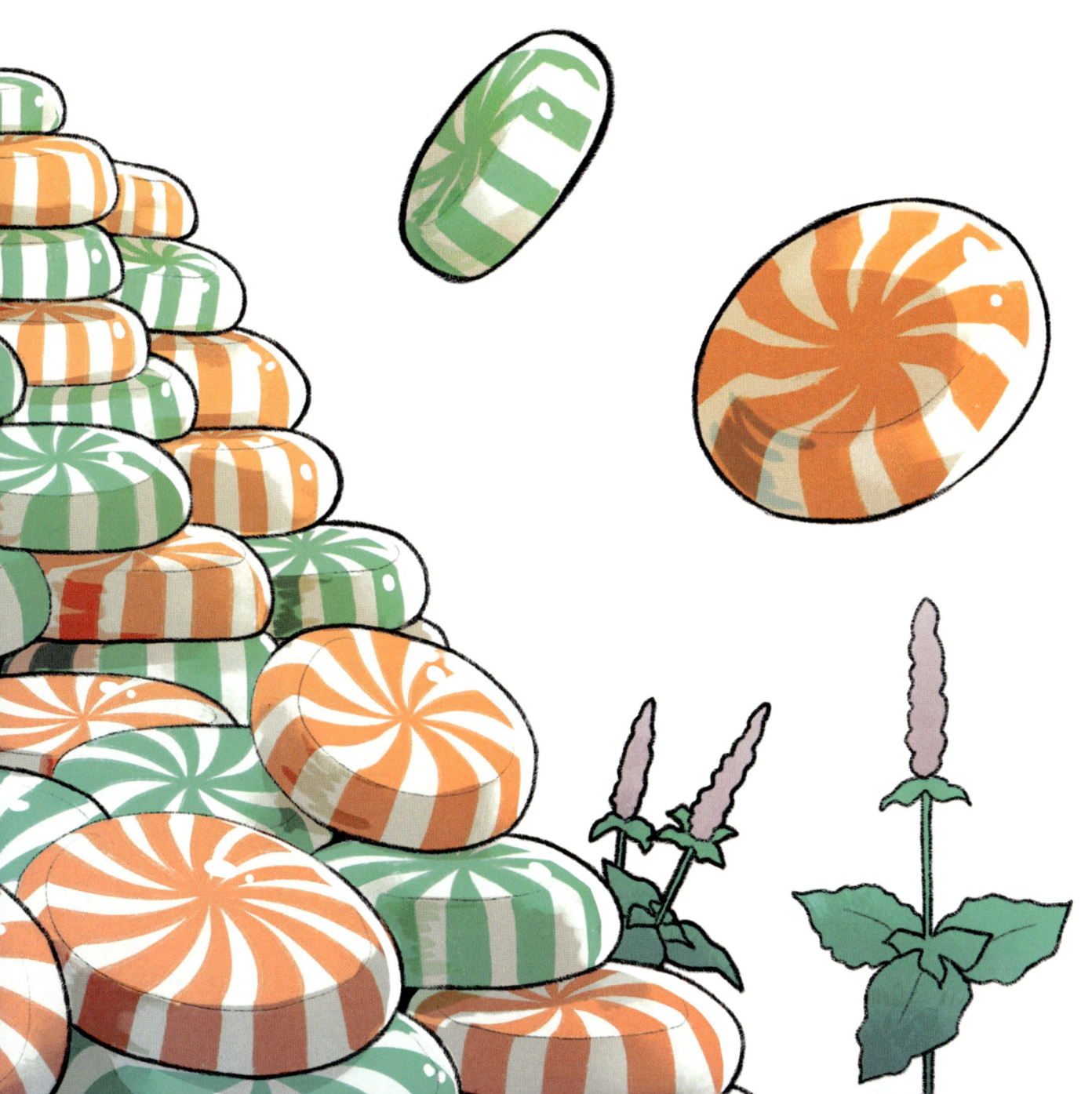

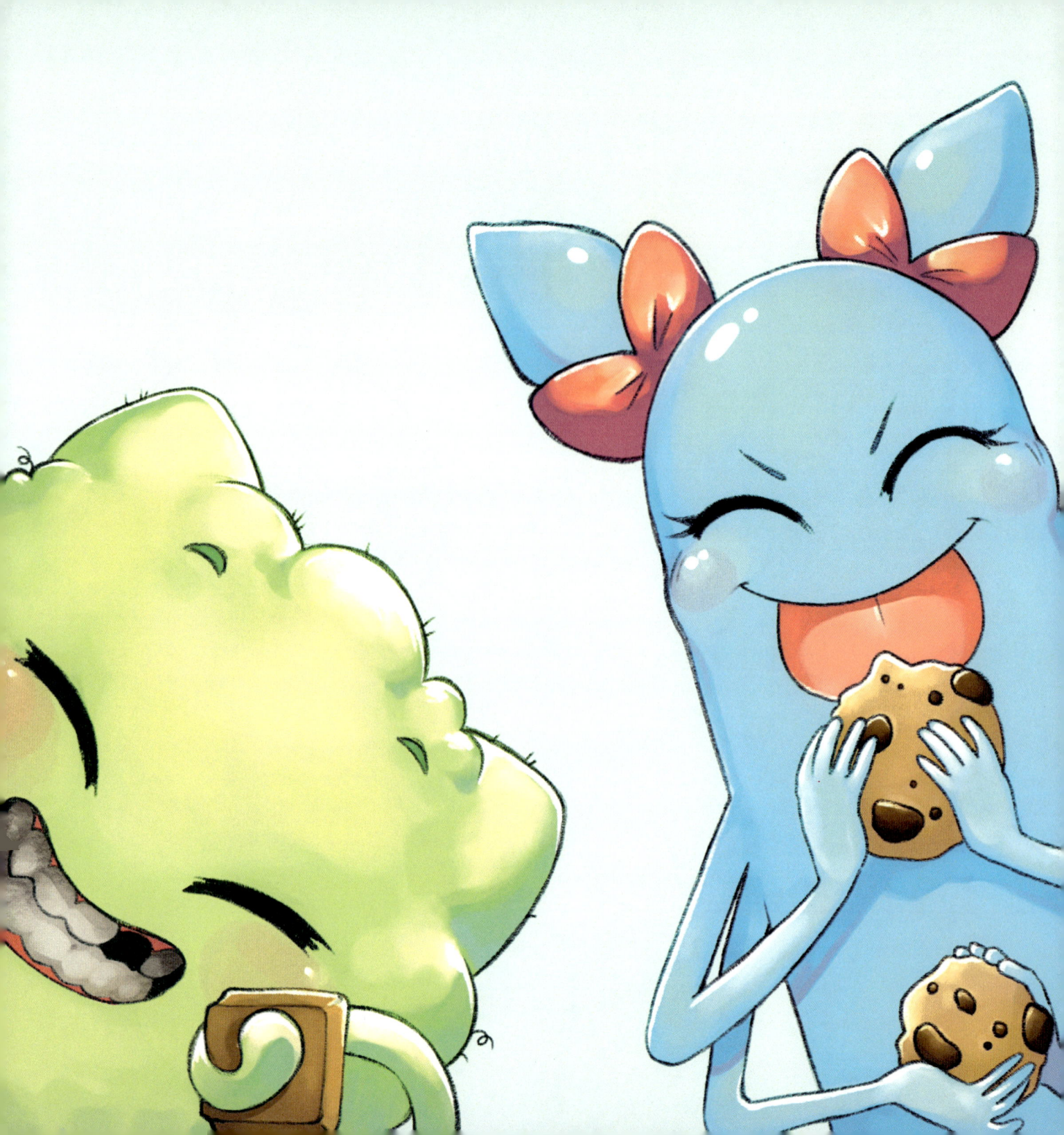

Candy?! Toothy and Mouthy perked up. They also loved sweets and started craving something tasty. Toothy found some leftover chocolate between the Betsy's teeth, and Mouthy spotted several cookie crumbs.

It's good that Betsy has not brushed her teeth! The monsters had never brushed their teeth, so their smiles were very black.

Before they ate their sweet supper, the monsters did not wash their hands and at the table they ate noisily and interrupted each other. They were very messy. Fortunately, today they did not throw food at each other, like they did yesterday. They had already grown a bit older and wiser during the day.

The little monsters had also learned new polite words, "Thank you! Everything was delicious." Perhaps they will grow up to be polite adult monsters after all!

After a hearty dinner, Toothy and Mouthy were full of energy and new ideas. There were still a lot of crumbs in the mouth.

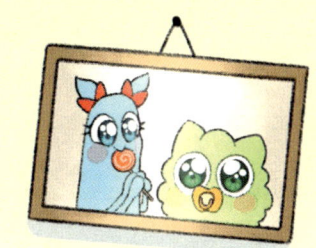

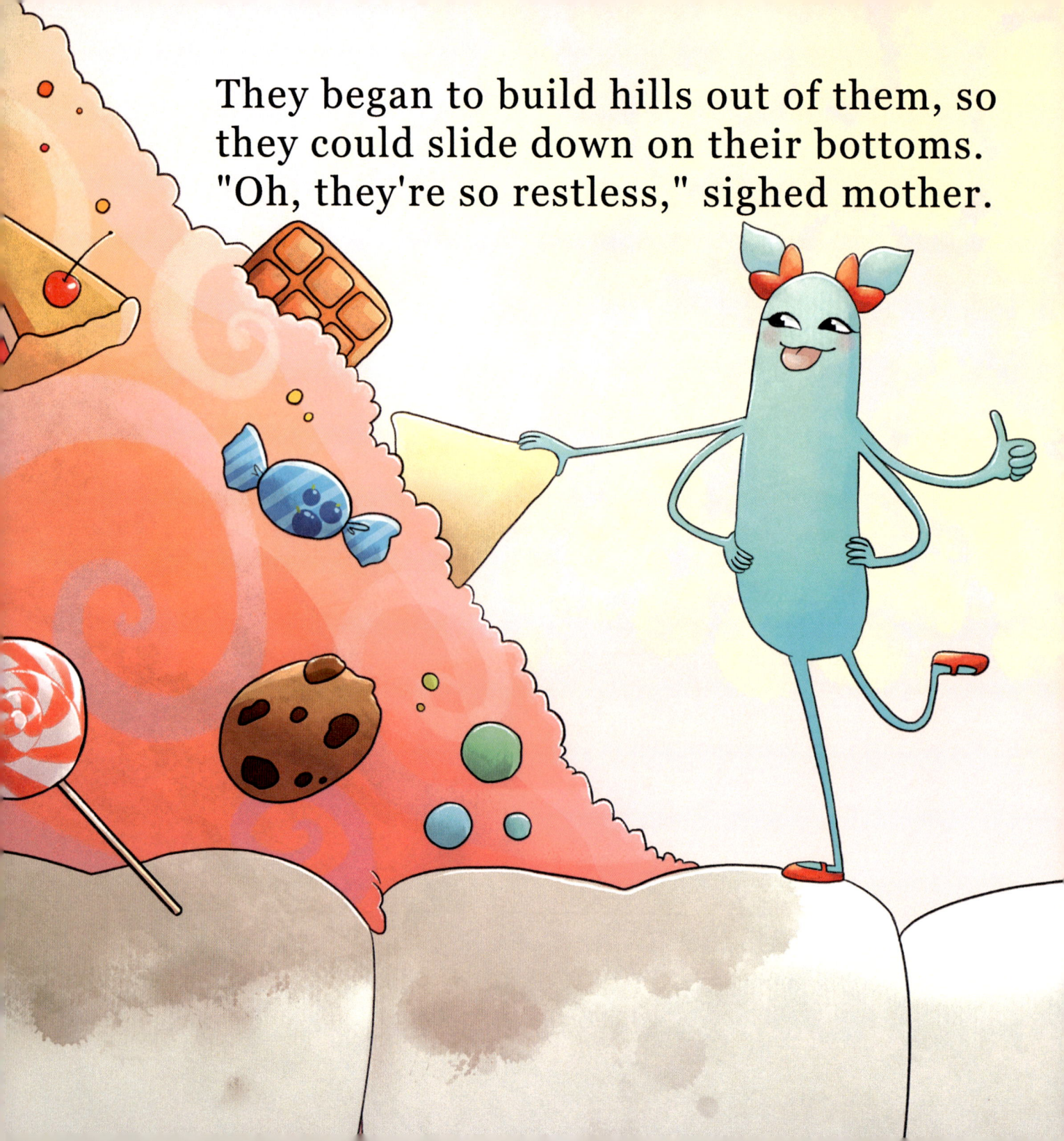

"If they don't go to bed, they will be building slides all night and under the sweet heaps your teeth will darken and start to decay."
"Mom, I know. That is called a cavity," Betsy said.

She had heard the word cavity in a toothpaste advertisement. It talked a lot about black spots and even holes in teeth, but, for some reason, it did not talk about the fact that cavities are caused by small monsters.

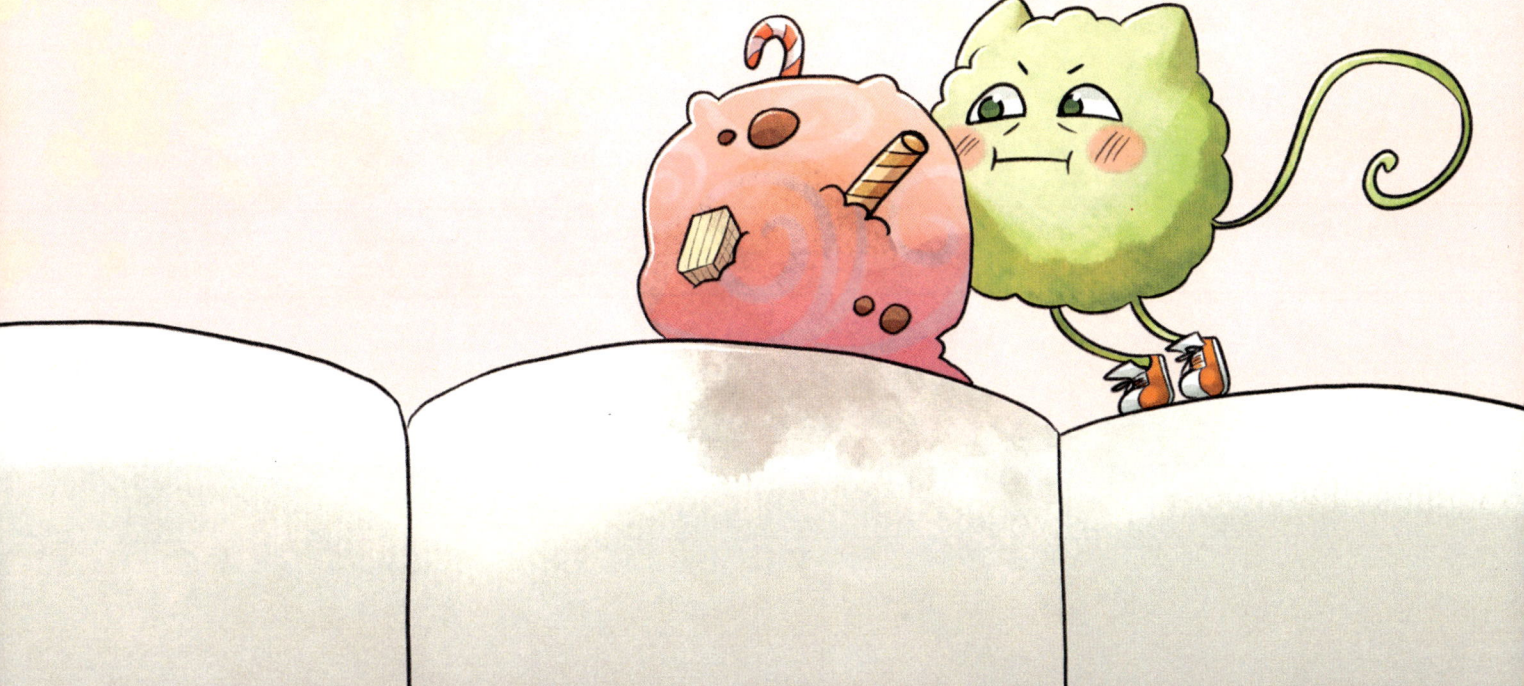

How can we get rid of these troublemakers? Betsy did not like to brush her teeth. Instead, she decided to drink some water to wash the monsters away once and for all.

Gulp! Gulp! A cool wave covered the monsters, but Toothy and Mouthy became even more excited. Now they began to splash and dive. They were not at all afraid of water, because their parents often took them to the swimming pool.

"How good your monsters are at swimming," mother said, looking at them amusing themselves.

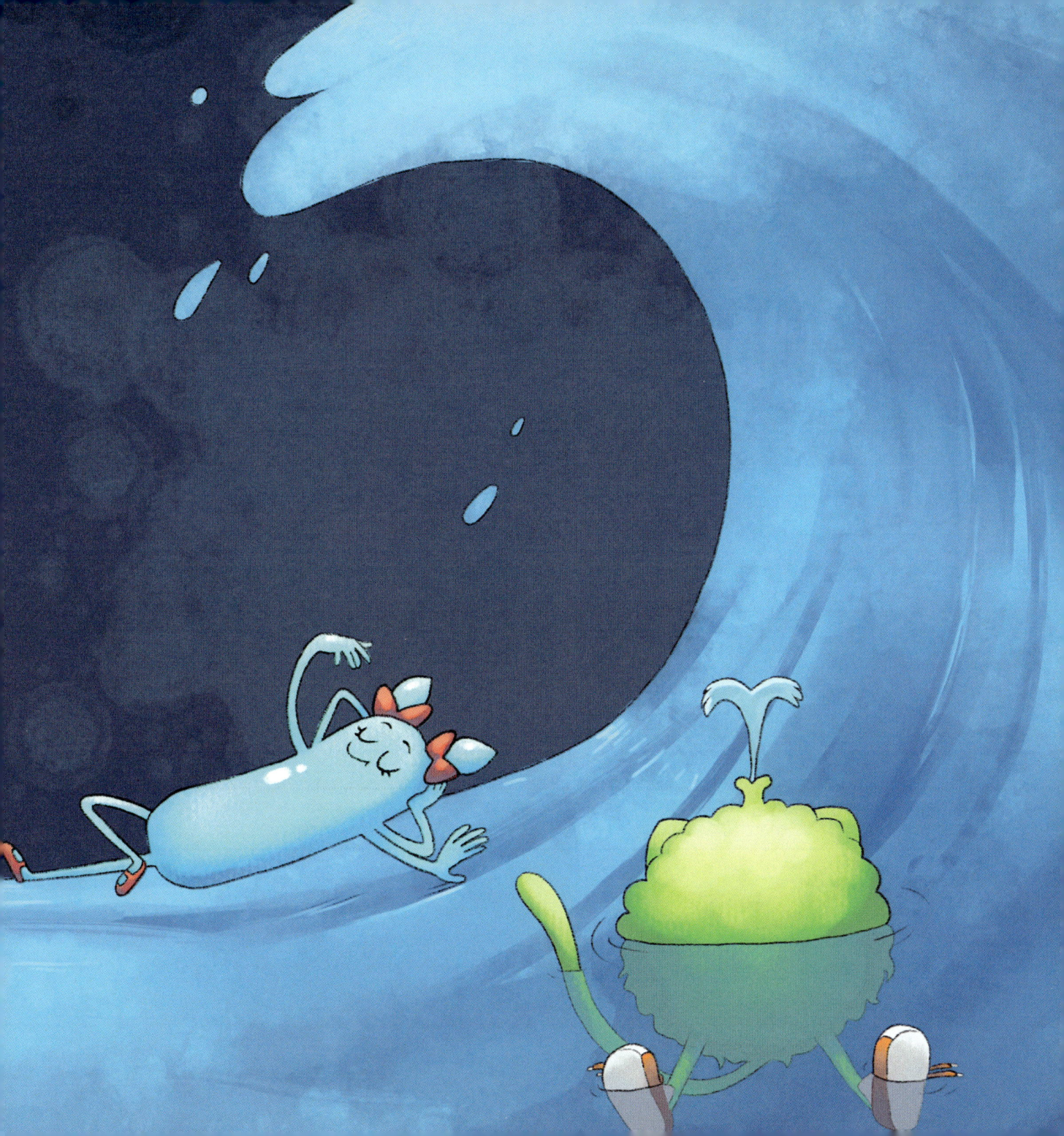

Toothy and Mouthy swam for so long that they began to get cold. Betsy felt them start to shiver and their teeth start to chatter. She felt sorry for the little monsters.

How could she warm them up?

"Let's make them a warm bath with bubbles," mother suggested. "They'll lie down in it, relax and quickly get sleepy."

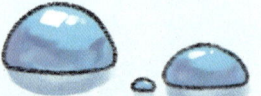

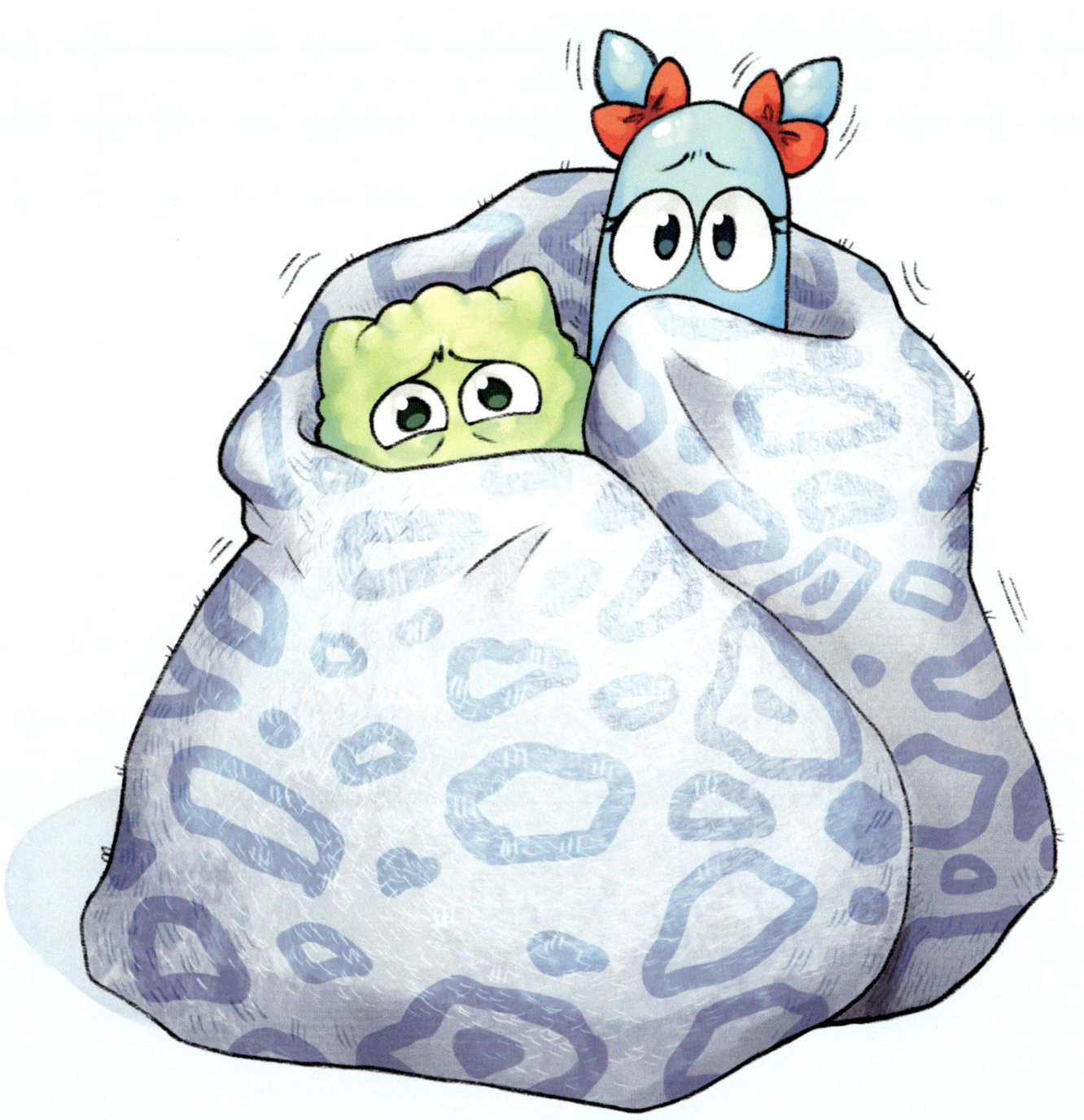

Betsy immediately agreed. Honestly, she was already getting quite tired herself. She made her little monsters a bubbly bath with strawberry-flavoured toothpaste.

While the monsters were laying in the sweet-smelling bath, Betsy stroked them with her toothbrush behind their ears, tickled their bellies and scratched their backs.

That's how the monsters became squeaky clean and everything in the mouth was put in order.

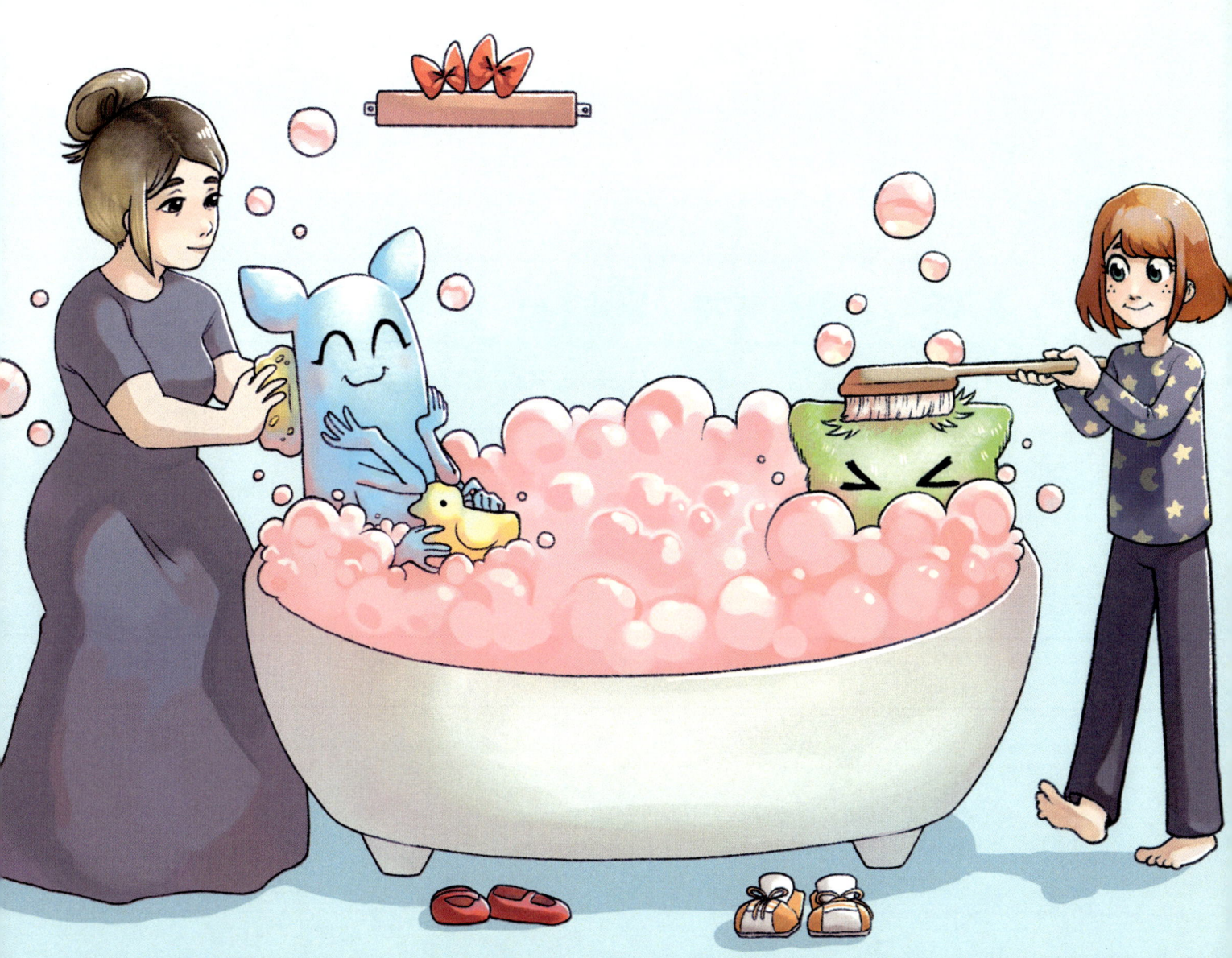

Mouthy was so sleepy that she barely made it to her bed. Little Toothy was fighting to keep his eyes open, but he wanted to play hide-and-seek with Betsy. He hid behind her upper teeth.

"Toothy, where are you? It's time to go to bed," Betsy called affectionately.

"We'll find him," mother smiled. "We have a device for finding disobedient monsters." She took out the floss.

They carefully threaded the floss between each of Betsy's teeth. Finally, they caught the little monster. He grasped the floss with his tail, his legs dangling in the air. Only now he realized that the time for play was over.

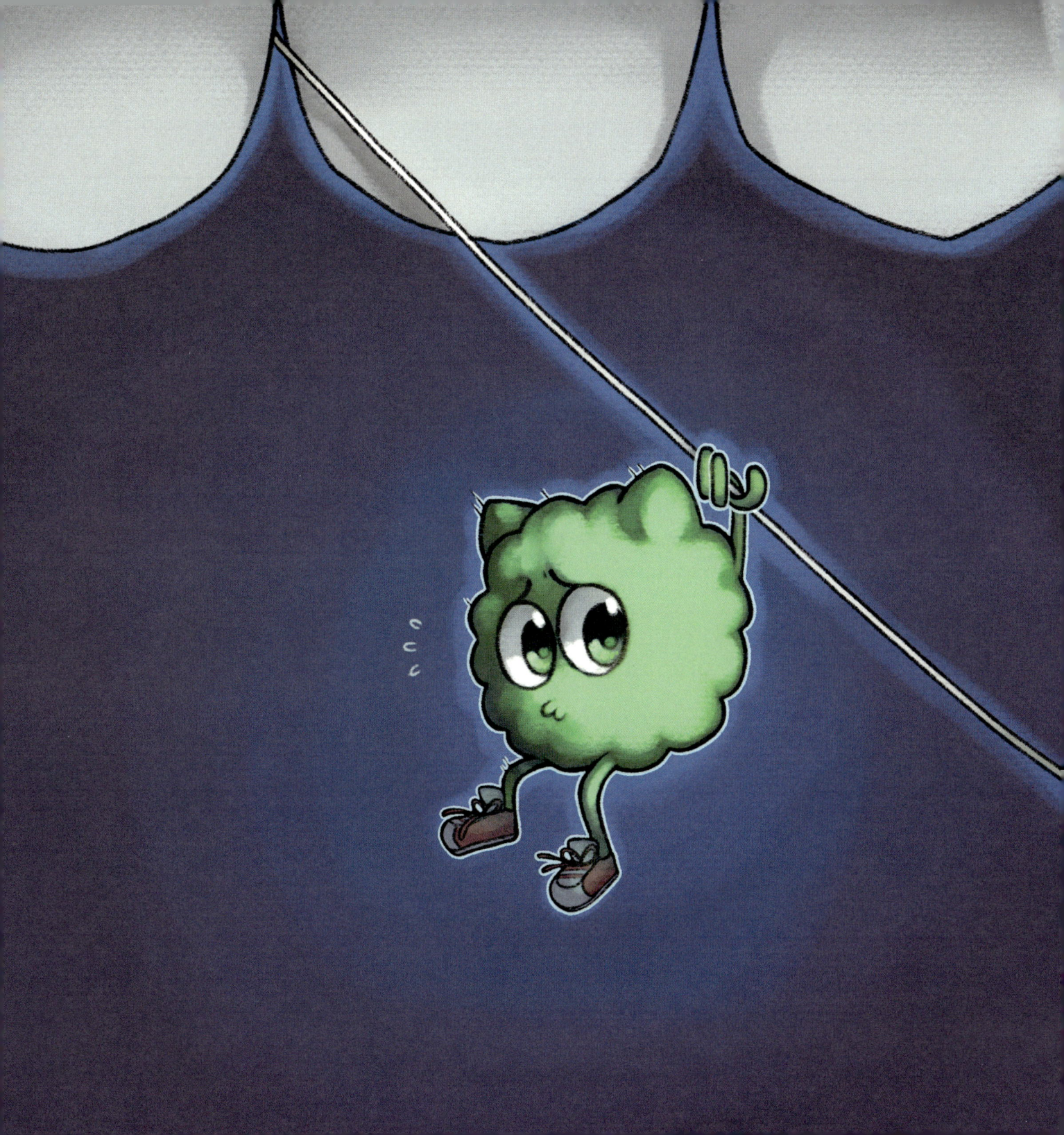

The monsters finally lay down to sleep. Their little beds were hidden under the tongue, where it was very warm and cozy. Now Toothy and Mouthy smelled so much of strawberries that mother's monsters completely forgot about mint candies and dreamed only of strawberries!

"Mummy, I love you so much! Even with your monsters," said Betsy, and gave mother a hug and kissed her on the cheek.

"I love you too! You're the best girl in the world!" mother replied.

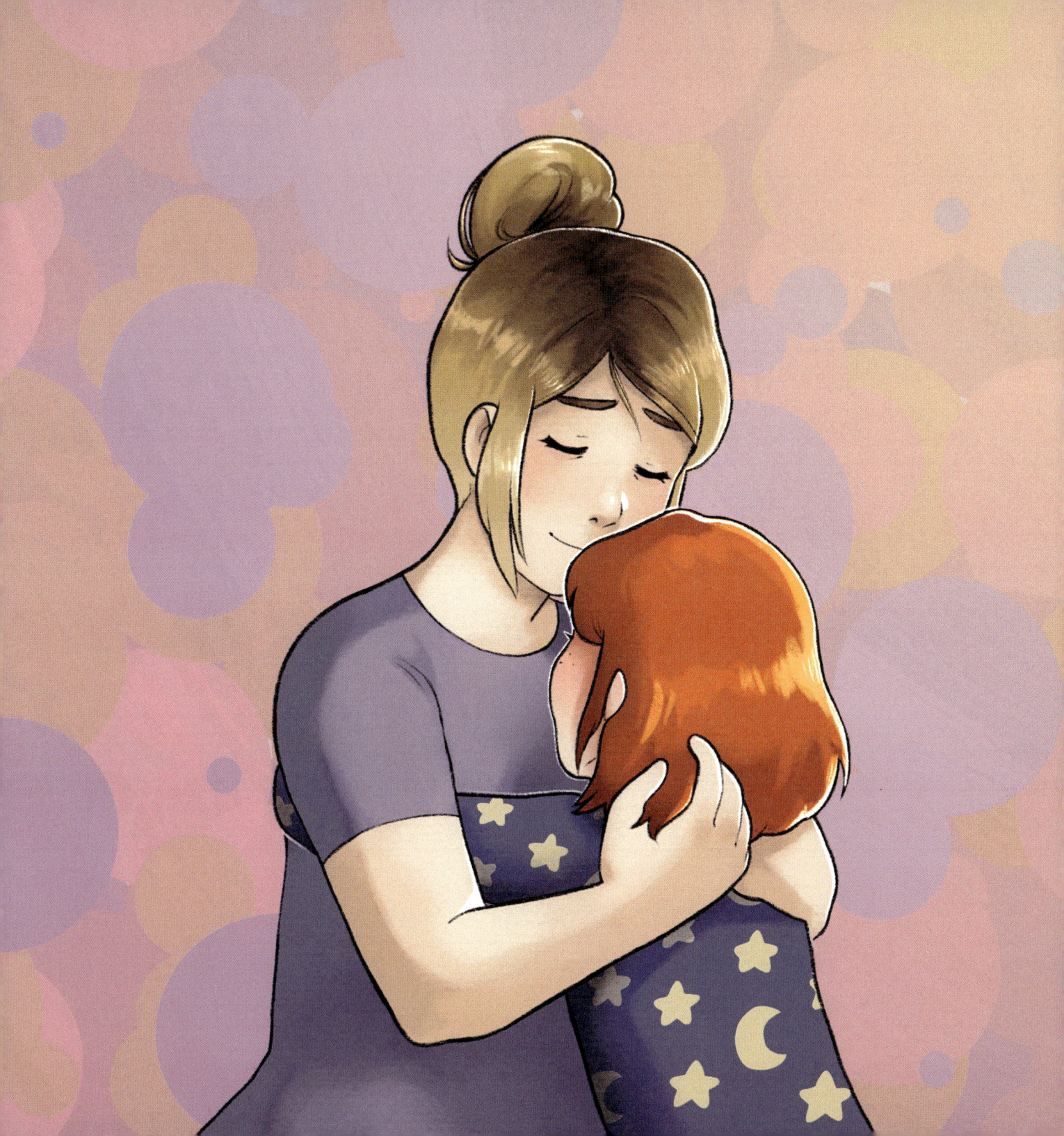

The little monsters, who had long been snoozing under the tongue, smiled in their sleep at the sound of such pleasant words.

They also loved their mothers very much, because for them they were also the best little monsters in the world!

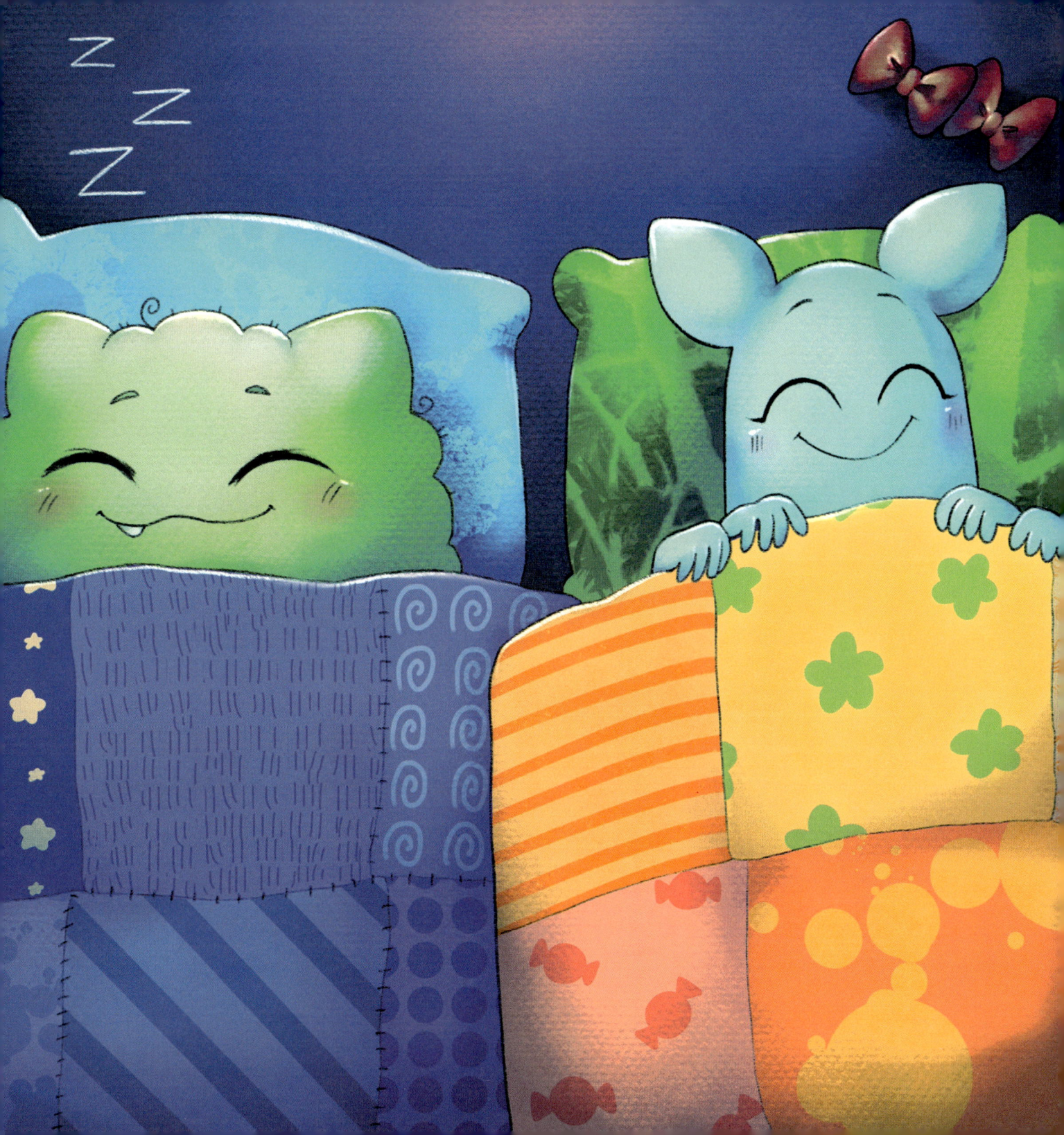

# Little monsters, it's time to go to bed!
## How to put little monsters to sleep with a toothbrush and dental floss

Written by Olivia Longray
Illustrated by Kristina Davtian

All rights reserved.
Text copyright @ Olivia Longray, 2018
Illustrations copyright @ Kristina Davtian, 2018
Translated by Jonathan Mahoney

ISBN: 9781726621014

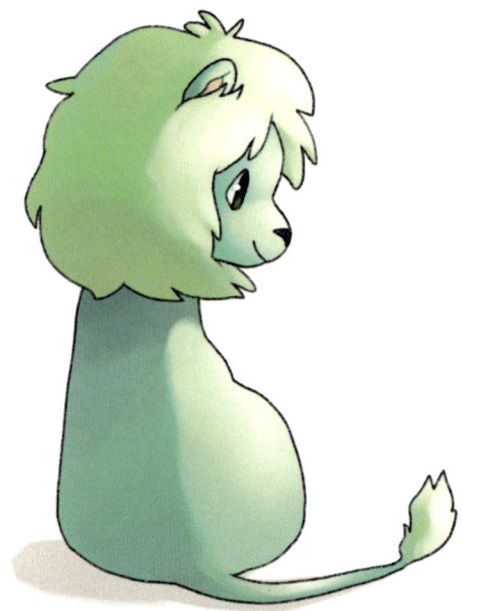
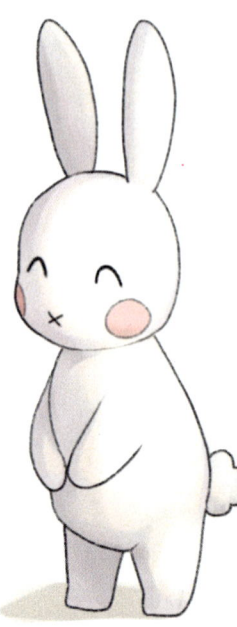

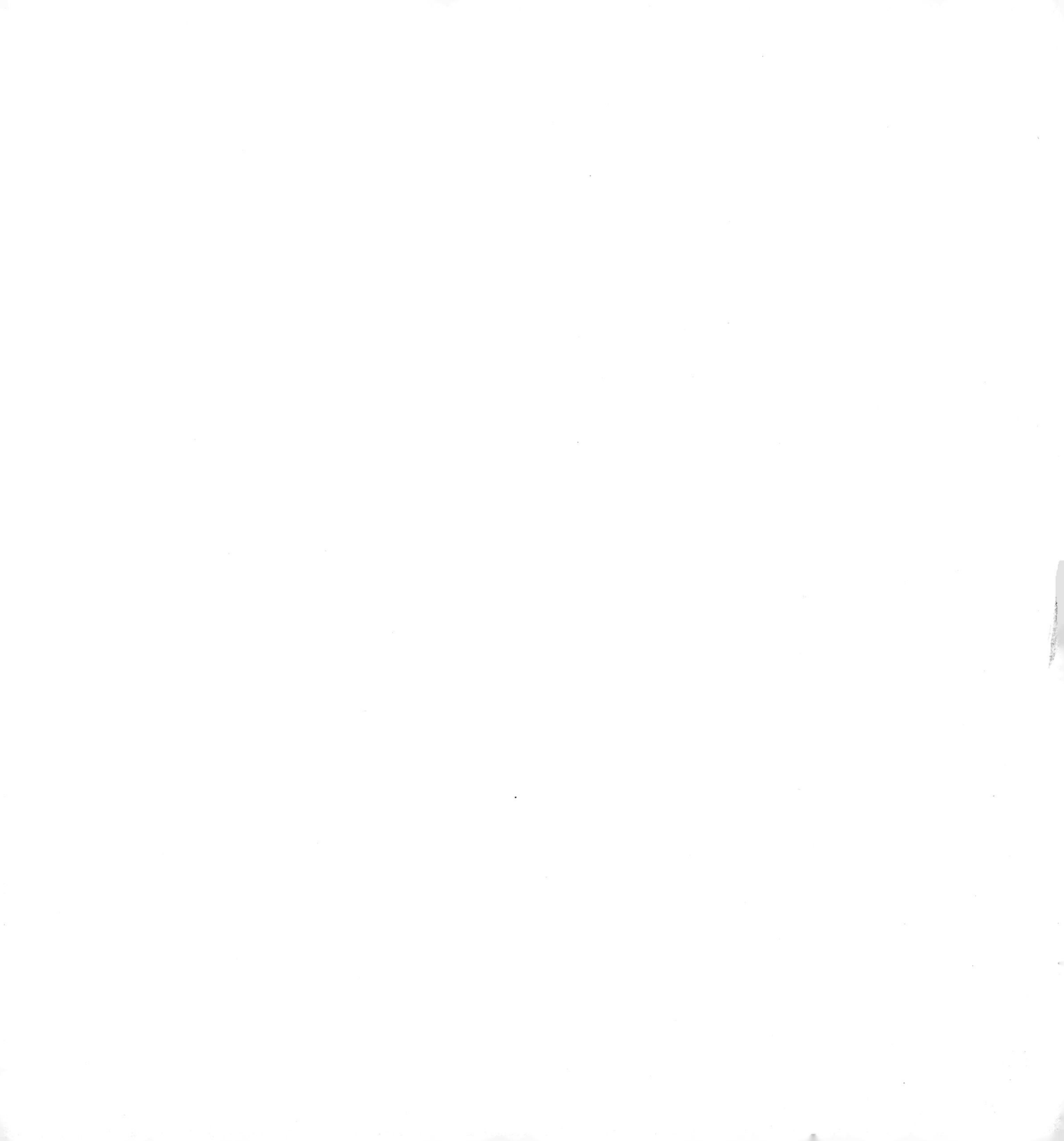

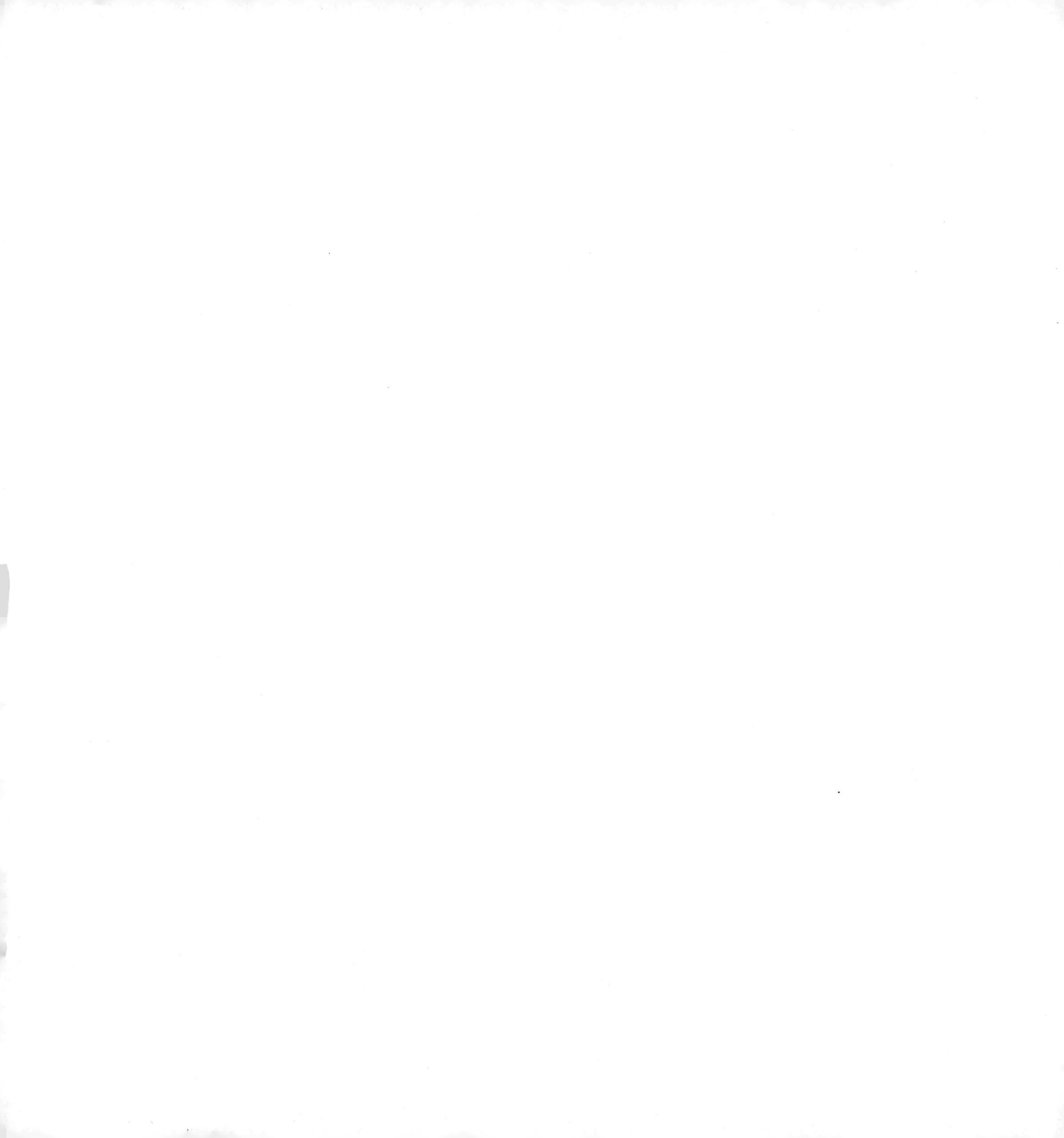